LIVING WITH HIV

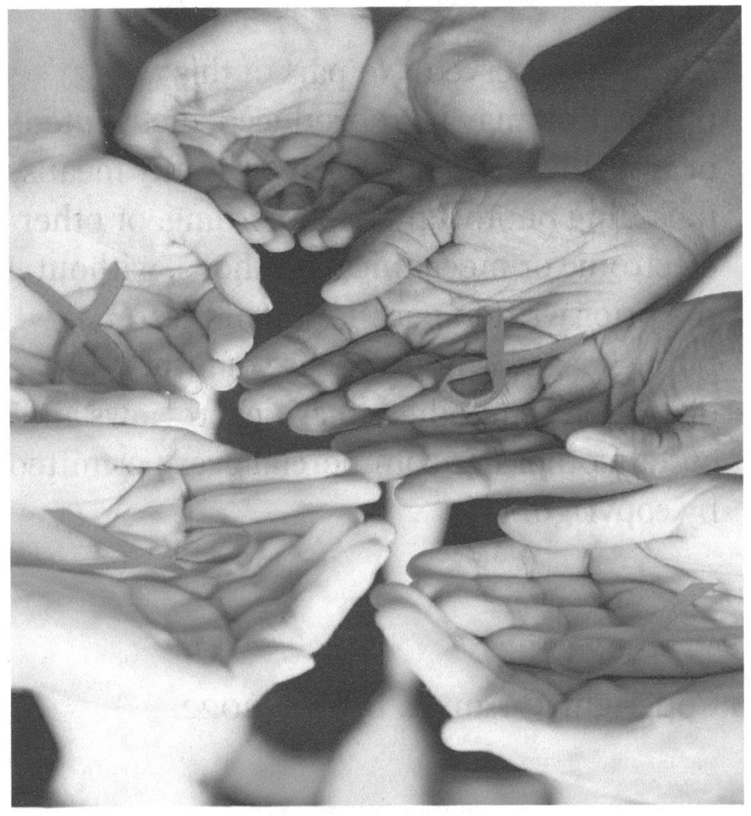

BATTLING DISCRIMINATION, STIGMA, AND DENIAL

Ann R. Brown

TABLE OF CONTENTS

DEFINING HIV: SYMPTOMS, WAYS OF TRANSMISSION AND PREVENTION

WHAT IS HIV?

Human immunodeficiency virus (HIV) is a virus that targets immune system cells, rendering an individual more susceptible to various illnesses and infections. It is shared by sharing injection equipment or through direct contact with the body fluids of an infected individual, most frequently during unprotected intercourse (sex without the use of a condom or HIV medication to prevent or treat HIV).

HIV can cause AIDS if not properly treated (acquired immunodeficiency syndrome). HIV cannot be eliminated by the human body, and no HIV treatment works. Therefore, if you have HIV, you will always have it.

SYMPTOMS OF HIV

For a very long period after becoming infected, people typically appear and feel in perfect health. For those who take HIV medications, the time it takes for any symptoms to appear might be 10 years or longer. Because of this, it's crucial to frequently be tested for HIV, especially if you've engaged in unprotected intercourse or shared needles. You can maintain your health with HIV therapy. Additionally, treatment can reduce or even eliminate your risk of transmitting HIV through intercourse.

You might experience fever, aches, and sickness for the first two to four weeks after becoming HIV-positive. Your body's initial response to the HIV infection is these flu-like symptoms. Since there is a lot of the virus in your system at this time, HIV transmission is quite simple. The symptoms only last a few weeks, and you often don't experience them again for years after that. However, HIV can still transmit to other individuals even if you don't feel well or have any symptoms.

Your immune system's CD4 cells, also known as T cells, are damaged by HIV. Your body has a difficult time fending off illnesses without CD4 cells. Because of this, you are more prone to develop severe infections from ones that otherwise wouldn't harm you. AIDS develops over time as a result of the harm HIV causes to your immune system.

HIV TRANSMISSION
- Sexual contact with an infected partner is the main way that HIV is transferred. During sexual intercourse, the virus enters the body via the lining of the vagina, vulva, penis, rectum, or mouth.

- HIV may also be transmitted via contact with blood that has been contaminated. The risk of contracting HIV via blood transfusions is very low because of the screening of blood for signs of HIV infection.

- Sharing needles, syringes, or other drug-use supplies with an HIV-positive person is a common way to transfer the infection. Through unintentional sticks with infected needles or other medical equipment, transmission from a patient to a healthcare worker or vice versa is very uncommon.

- HIV may also be passed from mother to child if the mother is infected and the child is nursed.

- Some bodily fluids cannot spread HIV. The following cannot transmit HIV:

- Saliva exchange, such as via closed-mouth kissing or the sharing of beverages or utensils

- Getting wet, sneezing, or crying into an HIV-positive person's tears

- Embracing, shaking hands, or touching communal items like silverware, cups, or toilet seats are examples of common physical contact.

- Water or air

- Because HIV can only be spread between people, pets, and insects (including mosquitoes) cannot transmit the virus and infect you.

HIV PREVENTION

It takes more than simply following the rules to avoid HIV. It is important to be aware of the hazards and comprehend how HIV is and is not spread. It involves going above and above to educate oneself on both cutting-edge and time-tested HIV prevention strategies. It mostly involves understanding oneself.

In the end, every individual is unique. Some persons are more prone to infection than others. Others may have particular objectives, such as beginning a family or becoming pregnant, which call for special thought and include various risks.

You must examine your risk factors honestly to protect yourself, and you must create a unique preventative plan to reduce the risks.

You could profit from employing one or more of these, depending on your particular risk factors:

- Condoms: Internal or external.
- Pre-exposure prophylaxis (PrEP) use in the absence of HIV.
- Maintaining an HIV-positive individual's undetectable viral load.
- Avoiding nursing if you have HIV and beginning HIV treatment while pregnant.
- Avoiding shared needles or syringes using PEP (post-exposure prophylaxis) if HIV was accidentally exposed.

Education is also important. The more protected you are, the more you will understand about HIV and how to prevent it.

PROGRESSION OF HIV TO AIDS

HIV infection spreads in phases and worsens without treatment. HIV steadily weakens the immune system, leading to acquired immunodeficiency syndrome in the end (AIDS).

HIV cannot be cured, although antiretroviral medication (often known as ART) may halt or stop HIV from progressing from one stage to the next. HIV medications make it possible for patients to live longer, healthier lives. To make a person's viral load undetectable is one of ART's primary objectives. A viral load test cannot identify an undetectable viral load, which indicates that the blood level of HIV is too low to be detected. The risk of HIV transmission to an HIV-negative partner during sex is almost zero for people with HIV who maintain an undetectable viral load.

The HIV infection process has three stages:

ACUTE HIV INFECTION: The initial stage of HIV infection is known as acute HIV infection, which typically appears 2–4 weeks after HIV infection.

Some individuals have flu-like symptoms at this time, including fever, headache, and rash. HIV multiplies quickly during the acute stage of infection and spreads all throughout the body.

The immune system's infection-fighting CD4 cells (CD4 T lymphocytes) are attacked and destroyed by the virus.

The risk of HIV transmission significantly rises during the acute HIV infection stage due to the very high HIV blood levels. If ART is started at this point, a person could benefit significantly in terms of their health.

CHRONIC HIV INFECTION: Chronic HIV infection is the second stage of HIV infection (also called asymptomatic HIV infection or clinical latency).

HIV continues to replicate in the body at this stage, but at extremely low levels. It's possible for people with persistent HIV infection to be symptom-free.

Without ART, chronic HIV infection typically progresses to AIDS in 10 years or more, while it may do so sooner in certain persons. The stage in which ART recipients may be may last for decades. While it is still possible to spread HIV at this stage, those who follow ART instructions to the letter and maintain an undetectable viral load essentially have no danger of passing the virus on to an HIV-negative partner via sex.

AIDS: The most advanced and dangerous stage of HIV infection. The immune system has been badly harmed by HIV, making it impossible for the body to resist opportunistic infections. People with HIV are diagnosed with AIDS if they have a CD4 count of less than 200 cells/mm3 or if they have specific opportunistic infections. Opportunistic infections are infections and infection-related cancers that occur more frequently or are more severe in people with weakened immune systems than in people with healthy immune systems. After receiving an AIDS diagnosis, a person may have a high viral load and be particularly likely to infect others with HIV. People with AIDS often live for three years without therapy.

GETTING DIAGNOSED

Human immunodeficiency virus (HIV), the virus that causes acquired immunodeficiency syndrome(AIDS), is most often diagnosed by blood testing. These exams search for antibodies to the virus that is present in infected people's blood. People who have been exposed to the virus need to get tested very away.

With HIV, early testing is essential. If you are HIV positive, you may create a treatment plan with your doctor to combat the disease and prevent consequences. Early testing might also warn you to stay away from risky conduct that can infect others.

Follow-up testing could be required since the development of antiviral antibodies can take anywhere between six weeks and six months. Your doctor will do a physical examination and inquire about your symptoms, medical history, and risk factors.

The following are the main exams used to identify HIV and AIDS:

ELISA TEST: HIV infection is discovered via the ELISA test, which stands for enzyme-linked immunosorbent assay. The Western blot test is often used to confirm the diagnosis if an ELISA test is positive. You should be tested again in one to three months if an ELISA test comes out negative but you believe you may have HIV. Because antibodies aren't created right away after infection, you may test negative for HIV for a window of a few weeks to a few months. ELISA is highly sensitive to chronic HIV infection. Even if your test results are negative within this time frame, you might still be highly infected with the virus and in danger of spreading the illness.

SALIVA TESTS: The inside of your cheek is rubbed with a cotton pad to collect saliva. The pad is put inside a vial and sent to a lab for analysis. In three days, the results will be released. A blood test should be used to verify positive findings.

The viral load test determines the level of HIV in your blood. In most cases, it's used to track the success of a medication or spot an early HIV infection. Reverse transcription polymerase chain reaction (RT-PCR), branched DNA (bDNA), and nucleic acid sequence-based amplification test are the three methods used to determine the HIV viral load in the blood (NASBA). These tests all operate on the same fundamental ideas. DNA sequences that bind particularly to those in the virus are used to identify HIV. It is important to remember that outcomes may differ across exams.

WESTERN BLOT: To verify a positive ELISA test result, a highly sensitive blood test is performed.

EMBRACING YOUR HIV STATUS: OVERCOMING DENIAL

Your whole world may abruptly alter if you are HIV positive. Who you tell, the healthcare professionals you choose, the way you manage your immune system, and how you wish to live with HIV are all important decisions.

Since 1981, more than 700,000 instances of AIDS have been documented in the US, and more than 900,000 people may now be living with HIV. It is reasonable to state that we are dealing with an epidemic, one that is most quickly spreading among minority and female groups. Learning about the disease's side effects and how they may impair your quality of life is only logical. Your HIV infection may have many side symptoms at once, just as with any other condition.

Although not all-inclusive, this list may include:

- Fatigue

- Anemia

- Digestion issues

- Bloating and Gas

- Diarrhea

- Lipodystrophy (body-form alterations)

- Elevated blood fat and sugar levels

- Skin Issues (e.g., rashes, dry skin, hair loss)

- Radicular Neuropathy

- Toxicity of the mitochondria

- Osteoporosis

- Osteonecrosis (bone death)

- Depression

BATTLING HIV DEPRESSION

With 22% of the population affected, clinical depression is the most prevalent mental health issue among those with HIV diagnoses. If you also misuse drugs or alcohol, this rate can be greater. Sadness and loss are common feelings after receiving an HIV diagnosis, but sadness and grief that progress to full-blown clinical depression are not seen as appropriate reactions. Depression may have a detrimental effect on your thoughts, feelings, body, and behavior. Additionally, it often remains misdiagnosed and untreated in HIV-positive people. The good news is that depression medications help patients better manage both illnesses,

just as substantial medical improvements
have helped HIV-positive people live fuller,
more productive lives. These therapies may
improve the quality of life and survival rates
for people with HIV and depression.

If you have been told you have HIV, you
should see the doctor often to keep the virus
under control. Your doctor and/or clinician
should do an annual mental health
evaluation in addition to physical exams and
testing. Since depression often coexists with
an HIV diagnosis, many patients may delay
seeking therapy because they believe it to be
a typical side effect of their condition.
Similar to this, many professionals neglect
to properly screen for depression in order to
respect the patient. But you should be aware
of the following indicators of depression:

- Overall negative attitude

- Loss of enjoyment or interest

- Suicidal ideas

- A sense of guilt

- Changes in appetite and weight

- Sleep disruption

- Issues with focus and attention

- Energy levels fluctuating and weariness

- Psychiatric-motor disorder

- Extreme pessimism or despair

- Ongoing agitation

- Affective instability is pronounced

- Unsuitable social behavior

- Feeling sluggish and slow

- Reduced sex desire

Treatment for depression is essential for HIV patients. Depression may make people with HIV stop taking their medications, stop coming to doctor's visits, and actively cease caring for themselves in general if it is not addressed. In addition, untreated sadness may result in riskier behavior such as drug and alcohol misuse as well as reckless actions that might expose people to HIV. Depression may result in suicide as well as a generalized bad quality of life, in addition to accelerating the progression of your HIV condition.

The good news is that there are treatments available to aid in your depression management, which may also enhance your HIV prognosis. Both medication and lifestyle adjustments have shown to be successful treatments for depression in people living with HIV.

The use of antidepressant drugs as a therapy for depression has been shown to be successful. Pay particular attention to any negative effects when taking antidepressants if you have HIV and are taking them. This is because there may be interactions between the antidepressants and other HIV-related drugs you are taking. Selective Seratonin Reuptake Inhibitors (SSRIs) and tricyclic antidepressants are the two types of antidepressants that are most often administered. Both have potential adverse effects, including diminished sexual function and desire, headaches, sleeplessness, exhaustion, irregular heartbeat, constipation, and upset stomach. Every medicine has to be taken under a doctor's supervision.

When you have been diagnosed with HIV, some lifestyle modifications have also been proved to be successful in treating depression. These include better sleeping patterns, psychotherapy, stress management, frequent exercise, and sun exposure. Acupuncture and massage have both been identified as effective complementary treatments for depression.

To maximize the effects of your treatments:

- Attend regular medical checks

- Maintain your HIV or depression drug regimen (unless advised by a doctor)

- Learn as much as you can about your disorders, depression and HIV, and get familiar with the warning signs and symptoms.

- Avoid using drugs and drinking.

- Attend therapy sessions often

- Be active.

DISCLOSING YOUR HIV STATUS

It may be unsettling and difficult to tell someone you are HIV positive, whether they are a close friend or a sexual partner. It's fair to be concerned about how they will respond or running into HIV stigma. However, it's crucial to have courage and speak up for both your sake and the sake of your loved ones.

Here are a few of my suggestions about how to approach the topic.

NOTIFYING RELATIVES AND FRIENDS

It might be tough to tell people you've known longer than you've known yourself that you have HIV, particularly when they're the ones who say they'll be there for you no matter what. How are you going to tell them? What if this is what makes their status in your life questionable? Although these are unsettling ideas, they are but that: ideas. The most devastating tales are often the ones we tell ourselves. They often have little to do with reality.

Although they have a reputation for being harsh critics of their loved ones who have HIV, parents, siblings, and other family members have also been known to stand up for them.

Here are some of my suggestions for telling loved ones that you have HIV:

- Wait until you are at ease. Be emotionally ready to disclose the knowledge before sharing it with others.

- When telling relatives and friends, be ready to answer their inquiries. They could be intimate and even

frightening. However, you could be
their sole source of HIV information.
No matter how their queries are
phrased, people desire to comprehend
what you come across. Answers
should be as brief and basic as
possible.

- No one, healthy or not, can
  successfully navigate through life
  alone. Additionally, everyone handles
  the illness differently. It may be a
  lonely journey at times, whether
  you've just received a diagnosis or
  have been living with HIV for some
  time.

- Having your loved ones close by either
  serve as a nice diversion or serve as a
  steady inspiration for you to keep
  going. The finest thing that can ever
  happen to you is teaching them how to
  be a member of your support system.

REVEALING IT TO A DATE OR PARTNER

It might be difficult to tell someone you're going to have sex with that you have HIV. Telling your friends and family might sometimes be easier.

However, in the U = U era, most experts agree that a virus with an undetectable viral load is not contagious. Despite the fact that most individuals are aware of this, some people may still feel hesitant or uneasy about having intercourse with an HIV-positive person.

When deciding whether to tell a partner about your positive status, bear the following in mind:

- Make sure you are informed.To respond, do as much research as you can about HIV treatments and safeguards.

- Support is reciprocal. Whether you intend to date them or not, get them to get checked and offer to accompany them.

- Whether you want to meet someone long-term or simply for a quick experience, it's crucial that you relax and communicate the facts if your sexual partners are aware of your situation.
- As though it is you who must hear it, imagine yourself in their position and reassure your date or partner in the manner in which you would want to be informed if it were the other way around.
- Ensure you maintain a healthy lifestyle, take your medicine as directed, and actively see a doctor.

Keep in mind that HIV is not a death sentence.

Consider it like this: Telling your intimate partner may either deepen your connection or prevent any future communication. Good if it draws you closer. Keep your attention on communication and observe the development of your connection. It's preferable to know this up front rather than discover it after you've spent time and energy into a relationship if they decide they no longer want to be associated with you after revealing.

Only when we give in to stigma does it have power. The response of your date or relationship is not always indicative of how everyone else will respond to your disclosure. There is someone out there who will like your sincerity and find your openness to be incredibly alluring.

THE LESSON

Nobody will respond the same when you disclose that you have HIV, thus there is no one optimal method to do it. However, telling your partner about your situation may also improve your bond and provide you with the support you didn't even realize you needed. It could become a little bit easier if you do your homework, are sincere, and are patient.

BATTLING DISCRIMINATION AND STIGMA

HIV STIGMA

HIV stigma refers to unfavorable perceptions of those who have the virus. The discrimination that results from classifying someone as a member of a group is what is deemed to be improper in society.

Here are a few illustrations:

- Believing that HIV can only be acquired by a specific group of people.

- Judging the moral character of those who take action to prevent HIV transmission.

- Belief that individuals deserve to contract HIV as a result of their decisions.

HIV DISCRIMINATION

Discrimination, on the other hand, refers to the actions brought on by stigmatizing attitudes or beliefs. HIV discrimination is the practice of treating persons who are HIV-positive and those who are not differently.

Here are a few illustrations:

- A medical practitioner declining to treat or assist an HIV-positive patient.

- Avoiding casual contact with an HIV-positive person.

- A community member becoming
  socially isolated because they have
  HIV.

- Using terms like "HIVers" or
  "Positives".

GETTING TREATMENTS

HIV TREATMENTS

Antiretroviral therapy (ART), a very successful drug used to treat HIV, is part of the HIV treatment regimen. Everyone with HIV is advised to start ART, and those who have been diagnosed with HIV should do so as soon as feasible, if not immediately.

A combination of HIV medications known as an HIV treatment regimen is used by those on ART. A person's first HIV treatment regimen typically consists of three HIV medications that must be taken precisely as directed from at least two separate HIV drug classes. Numerous solutions combine two or three distinct HIV medications into a single once-daily tablet. If your doctor believes you satisfy specific criteria, you may also be allowed to get long-acting HIV medication injections every two months.

How Important Is HIV Treatment?

If taken as directed, HIV medication lowers your viral load, or how much HIV is present in your blood, to a very low level, which maintains your immune system functioning and helps you stay healthy. Viral suppression is the presence of fewer than 200 HIV copies per milliliter of blood.

HIV medications may potentially reduce your viral load to a point where a routine lab test is unable to detect it. An undetectable amount of viral load is what this is. Most people may attain an undetectable viral load within 6 months of commencing therapy if they take HIV medications as directed.

Many individuals will rapidly reduce their viral load to undetectable levels, however, a small percentage of those newly beginning HIV medication may need additional time.

The viral load should be kept as low as feasible for crucial health reasons. Living a long and healthy life with HIV is possible for those who are aware of their status, take their HIV medication as directed, and achieve and maintain an undetectable viral load.

A significant preventive benefit is also seen. When taking their HIV medications as directed and maintaining an undetectable viral load, people with HIV cannot sexually transfer the virus to their HIV-negative partners. Find out more about the advantages of having an undetectable viral load for prevention.

When you are dedicated to taking your medications precisely as directed and are aware of what to anticipate from your HIV treatment, it is most likely to be effective. You may better understand HIV and manage it by working with your healthcare physician to create a treatment plan.

HIV will target your immune system if you don't get treatment, which may lead to the emergence of many malignancies and life-threatening diseases. You are more susceptible to contracting an opportunistic infection if your immune system is compromised. These infections may affect individuals who aren't receiving treatment and whose immune systems have been compromised by HIV, even though they typically don't harm people with healthy immune systems. To stop certain infections, your doctor could recommend medications.

When Should HIV Treatment Begin?

No matter how long you've had the virus or how healthy you are, it's critical to begin HIV medication therapy as soon as you are diagnosed if you have the disease. HIV medication may prolong your life and decrease the spread of the virus.

Starting HIV medications as soon as possible is crucial for persons with HIV who have an early HIV infection or a condition that defines AIDS. Early HIV infection is defined as the first six months after HIV infection.

If they are not already taking them, people with HIV who get pregnant should begin taking HIV medications as soon as possible to preserve their health and stop HIV from being passed on to the unborn child.

Speak to your doctor about the advantages of starting treatment if you have been diagnosed with HIV but are not already taking HIV medications.

Are there side effects from HIV treatment?

HIV medications may have negative effects on certain patients, just as other medications do. But not everyone encounters them. The HIV medications being used now are less potent and have fewer adverse effects than in the past. Each form of HIV medication has potential side effects that might vary depending on the patient. Once you start taking a medication, certain side effects may appear and may only last a few days or weeks. Other adverse effects may not manifest for a longer time.

The HIV medication side effects that are most often reported include:

- Nausea and diarrhea

- Diarrhea

- Trouble sleeping

- Mouth ache

- Headache

- Rashes

- Dizziness

- Fatigue

Additionally, women and men may have distinct adverse effects from HIV medications.

Before you skip any doses or stop taking the medication, see your doctor or pharmacist if you encounter side effects that are severe or cause you to want to stop taking your HIV treatment.

Drug resistance may develop by skipping doses or abruptly beginning and stopping HIV medication, which is bad for your health and restricts your choices for further treatment. Your doctor can consider switching your HIV medications to another kind that might be more effective for you to lessen or eliminate adverse effects.

Should You Continue HIV Treatment?

Yes. You must continue taking your HIV medicines as directed since ART is not a cure and the virus still lives in your body even if your viral load is undetectable. Your viral load will soon increase if you stop taking your HIV medication.

Speak with your healthcare practitioner right away if you have stopped taking your HIV medication or if you are having problems taking all the dosages as directed. Up till your viral load is determined to be undetectable once again, your doctor can assist you to get back on track and go through the ideal methods for preventing HIV transmission to your sexual partners.

What Is Drug Resistance for HIV?

HIV multiplies quickly when HIV isn't completely under control by HIV medication. HIV may sometimes mutate (change form) when it multiplies in the body, creating new viral strains that might not be as responsive to a certain medication as the original virus was. The term for this is drug resistance.

HIV medications that formerly managed a person's HIV are no longer effective against newly developed, drug-resistant HIV. In other words, HIV medications are unable to stop the spread of HIV that is resistant to treatment. HIV therapy might be unsuccessful due to drug resistance.

A person may acquire drug-resistant HIV at the outset of their infection or after commencing HIV medications. HIV that is drug-resistant may potentially transfer from one person to another. Drug-resistance testing determines which HIV medications if any, won't work against your particular strain of the virus. The findings of drug-resistance testing assist in selecting the HIV medications to be used in an HIV treatment plan.

Following the directions on your HIV medication may help avoid drug resistance.

ACCEPTING LIFE WITH HIV: MOVING FORWARD

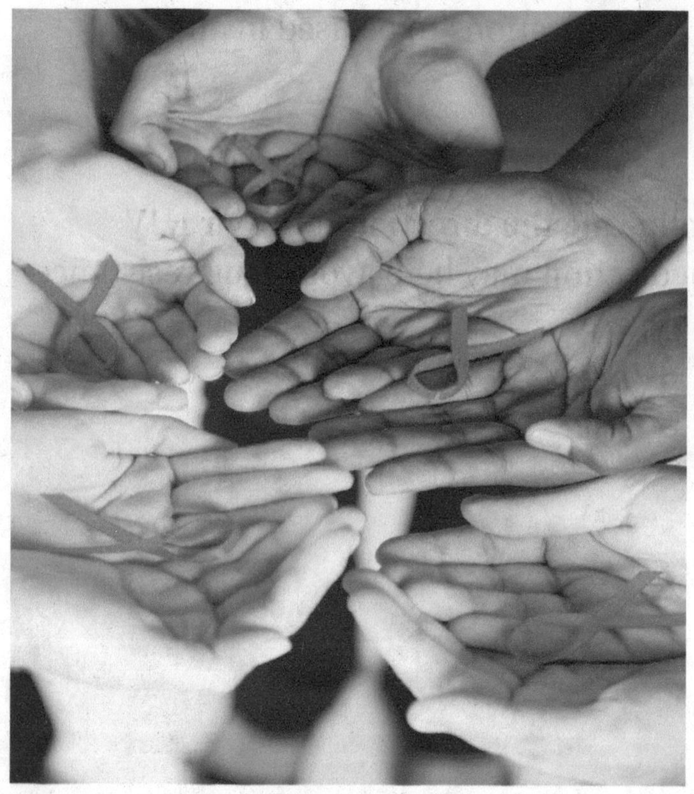

After receiving an HIV diagnosis, life does not end. Actually, given the right care, individuals with HIV often have long, healthy lives. Similar to diabetes or heart disease, HIV may be a chronic, controllable condition. You can manage HIV by looking after your general health:

- Daily medication intake.

- Regularly see the dentist and the doctor.

- Eat a balanced diet.

- Avoid smoking and using recreational drugs when exercising frequently.

- Don't drink too much.

- When having sex, use condoms (it can protect others from getting HIV, prevent unintended pregnancy, and

protect you from other sexually
transmitted diseases).

HIV affects millions of individuals, so you're
not alone. The majority of individuals have
an STD at least once in their lives, thus
having HIV or another STD is nothing to be
embarrassed or ashamed of. You're not
"filthy" or a horrible person because of it.

It may be quite unpleasant to learn you have
HIV. At first, you can feel angry, humiliated,
terrified, or embarrassed. But as time
passes, you'll probably start to feel better
since obtaining therapy and having a strong
support network are incredibly helpful.

www.ingramcontent.com/pod-product-compliance
Lightning Source LLC
Chambersburg PA
CBHW012312240726
48656CB00008B/2652